Nutrition and Fitness for Mental Well-being

Table of Contents

Chapter 1. Introduction

Unveiling our Special Report: Nutrition and Fitness for Mental Wellbeing! Traverse through this fun and relatable journey, where inspiring tales meet scientific truths to shed light on two fundamentals reflecting our mental stamina - nutrition and fitness. Tempting isn't it? We promise you an enlightening expedition, unearthing the profound impact what you eat and how you move can make on your mental state. Ready to enhance your cognitive sharpness, dispel stress, boost moods and embrace happiness? Dive headfirst into our meticulously compiled report and let's start making those mentally nourishing lifestyle choices now! Get ready to feed your mind and body with rich information that aligns perfectly with your pursuit of a happier, healthier life! What are you waiting for? Adventure into the invigorating realm of mindful living awaits in our uniquely curated report - expert knowledge made enjoyable!

Chapter 2. The Intricate Link between Nutrition, Fitness and Mental Health

Healthy sustenance and an active lifestyle unequivocally hold sway over our mental state. Let's embark on this enlightening exploration to appreciate how nutrition, exercise, and mental well-being are closely intertwined.

2.1. The Biochemistry of Foods

The nutrients we derive from food influence various bodily processes, including those that govern our mood and brain function. Essential brain chemicals, or neurotransmitters, like serotonin, dopamine, and norepinephrine, are directly regulated by what we eat.

Serotonin, known as the 'happy chemical,' regulates mood, emotional well-being, and sleep. It is synthesized from tryptophan, an essential amino acid obtained from food. Tryptophan is prevalent in high-protein foods like turkey, eggs, cheese, fish, and nuts. Consuming these foods can substantially enhance the serotonin levels in the brain, thus prompting a sense of calm and happiness.

Dopamine, referred to as the 'feel-good neurotransmitter,' controls our brain's reward and pleasure centers and helps regulate emotional responses. Dopamine synthesis necessitates the intake of amino acids phenylalanine and tyrosine found in protein-rich foods, such as dairy, eggs, meat, and certain plant-based foods, including apples, bananas, beetroot, and leafy greens.

Norepinephrine, aiding focus and alertness, is derived from dopamine. Its production can be boosted through a diet rich in tyrosine-containing foods. Moreover, the benefits of a balanced Omega-3 and Omega-6 fatty acid intake cannot be overstated. These fatty acids form an integral part of nerve cells and help modulate mood and cognitive function. Seafood, walnuts, almond, flax seeds, and chia seeds are standout sources of Omega-3s.

This crucial relationship between nutrients and brain function emphasizes the imperative need for a balanced diet suffused with protein, healthy fats, complex carbohydrates, and fiber, along with essential vitamins and minerals.

2.2. Fitness and Brain Chemistry

Now, pivoting towards fitness, let's dissect how exercise influences your mental well-being. When you engage in physical activities, your body releases endorphins, often termed 'natural painkillers' or 'feel-good hormones.' These chemicals interact with the receptors in your brain, reducing the perception of pain and triggering a positive feeling in the body, similar to that produced by morphine.

The reduction in anxiety and improvement in mood post-exercise underpin the 'runner's high' theory. Besides endorphin secretion, exercise also stimulates the production of serotonin, dopamine, and norepinephrine, contributing to mood enhancement and improved cognitive function.

Exercise also triggers the growth of new brain cells and facilitates neural plasticity, thereby improving memory, attention, and overall brain health. It fosters sound sleep and alleviates stress, all crucial for maintaining psychological well-being.

2.3. Dietary Recommendations for Brain Health

Let's shift our focus to some dietary recommendations that can bolster your mental health:

1. Eating a balanced diet with a healthy mix of fruits, vegetables, lean proteins, whole grains, and healthy fats is pivotal.

2. Adequate hydration is necessary for cognitive function; consuming approximately 2 liters of water daily can keep hydration levels optimal.

3. Cut down on refined sugars and processed foods, as these have been linked to inflammation and oxidative stress, potentially leading to mental health issues.

4. Opt for foods rich in antioxidants, such as berries, nuts, whole grains, and green vegetables to combat oxidative stress.

5. Ensure an adequate intake of prebiotics found in whole grains, bananas, onions, garlic, and other foods to help maintain a healthy gut, as some mental health problems have been linked to gut health issues.

2.4. Exercise Recommendations for Mental Health

Now, let's list some fitness guidelines that can fortify your psychological well-being:

1. Incorporate at least 30 minutes of moderate-intensity exercise like brisk walking most days of the week.

2. Including aerobic exercises in your routine can elevate cardiovascular fitness and boost endorphin levels.

3. Strength training exercises a few times a week can enhance muscle tone, metabolic rate, and mood.

4. Engage in flexibility exercises such as yoga and Pilates to improve joint health, reduce stress, and promote mood stability.

5. Consider mindful exercises like Tai Chi or Qigong to foster harmony between the mind and body, enhancing cognitive function and overall well-being.

2.5. Tying Nutrition and Fitness Together for Mental Well-being

Healthy nutrition and regular exercise are integral to mental well-being. Consuming a balanced diet enhances the neurotransmitter production that regulates mood while keeping the gut healthy. Simultaneously regular exercise induces chemical changes in the brain that foster relaxation, enhance mood, and improve cognitive function. Together, they create synergistic benefits for our mental health, underscoring the imperative need to make healthful food choices and to stay active.

Never forget – you are what you eat, and how you move shapes your mental agility. Switch to healthier food options, weave in regular exercise, and experience how it impacts your mental state. You'd be surprised at something so fundamental exhibiting such remarkable power!

Nutrition, fitness, and mental health are interconnected strands in the fabric of overall wellness. Prioritize them to unravel a happier, healthier self. Hold this guide close to your heart, let it steer you towards a mindful journey of nourishing your mind and body most beneficially. With every mindful bite and every determined stride, celebrate the grandeur of a healthful life!

Remember, the journey to mental well-being is an inward journey. It begins with you deciding to take that first step towards conscious, healthful living. And on this journey, we hope that this guide proves to be a supportive companion – enriching not just your understanding but also inspiring you to unfold layers of a fitter, happier, healthier self.

Chapter 3. Essential Nutrients: Fuel for the Mind

Our bodies, like intricate machines, require a wide variety of nutrients to function at their peak. They are the building blocks of life, supplying us with the energy to carry out essential processes, aiding in the repair and growth of tissues, and enabling our bodies to function optimally. Just as a car needs fuel to run, our brains need nutrients to work effectively too. Let's dive deep and know about these nutritional superheroes that act as the 'fuel' for our mind!

3.1. The Brain: A Power-Hungry Organ

The brain, although only constituting approximately 2% of our total body weight, consumes approximately 20% of our daily energy intake. Our brain, being a complex and energy-consuming organ, requires a constant supply of nutrients for its optimal performance.

3.2. Macronutrients – Breaking Down the Big Three

Macronutrients are nutrients that the human body requires in large amounts. They consist of carbohydrates, proteins, and fats.

Carbohydrates

Carbohydrates are the primary source of energy for our bodies and brain. When we eat carbohydrates, our bodies convert them into glucose, which can be used immediately for energy or stored for later use.

Proteins

Protein, the body's building block, also plays a crucial role in the health of the brain. Our brains use amino acids (the building blocks of proteins) to produce neurotransmitters. For instance, the brain uses the amino acid tryptophan to produce serotonin, a neurotransmitter associated with mood regulation.

Fats

Despite its bad reputation, fat is a crucial component of a healthy diet. Particularly, unsaturated fats are critical for brain health. They make up a significant portion of the brain tissue and are essential for cognitive functions such as learning and memory.

3.3. Micronutrients and Brain Health

Nourishing the brain isn't solely about macronutrients. Several micronutrients, such as vitamins and minerals, also play a vital role.

Vitamin B complex

The B vitamins, including B6, B9, and B12, are essential for the brain's healthy function, playing a major role in producing energy and neurotransmitters.

Vitamin D

Typically known for its role in bone health, Vitamin D is also associated with cognitive health. Research has found links between vitamin D deficiency and cognitive decline.

Minerals

Certain minerals such as iron, magnesium, and zinc are known for their impact on brain function. Iron, for example, is essential for delivering oxygen to the brain, whereas magnesium and zinc are involved in several neurological pathways.

3.4. Hydration Matters

Water makes up about 75% of the brain's weight and plays a crucial role in maintaining overall brain health, helping in cognitive functions and mood regulation. Staying hydrated is essential for maintaining mental alertness and reducing the risk of cognitive decline.

3.5. Influence of Diet on Mood and Mental Health

Understanding the impact of nutrients on our body is one thing, acknowledging their major role in mood regulation and mental health is another. Various studies indicate that a well-balanced diet can reduce the risk of depression, anxiety, and ADHD among others.

3.6. Role of Gut Health in Mental Well-being

Recent research stresses the importance of gut health on mental well-being. The gut-brain axis, a communication network between our gut and brain, can influence our mental health. Thus, a diet that encourages a healthy gut microbiome can potentially improve our mental health.

Achieving 'Nutrition Excellence' can seem like a lofty goal. Yet, it is not as formidable as it might initially appear. As we delve deeper into understanding the role of nutrition in mental health, it becomes evident that our daily choices significantly influence our mental well-being. Armed with the right information and conscious decision making, we can chart a course towards a richer, healthier mental landscape. The journey to mental wellness begins at our dining tables – breakfast, lunch, dinner, and every nourishing snack in between!

Remember, the key here is balance and moderation. Achieving your best brain health doesn't mean significantly altering your diet overnight or embarking on aggressive detox programs. Instead, it means making consistent, healthful choices daily - nourishing your body and mind for the long haul. Here's to smart eating for a healthy mind!

Chapter 4. Workout Your Way to Positivity: Exercise and Mood Enhancement

Stress, depression, and anxiety, the consistent villains of our modern age, have the potential to dismantle our psychological equilibrium. A potent weapon within our reach to combat these menacing mental health issues, surprisingly or unsurprisingly to some, is regular exercise. Often underestimated, physical fitness goes far beyond just shaping your physique; it substantially contributes to creating a healthier and happier mind.

4.1. The Science behind Exercise and Mood Enhancement

Exercise is not just about aerobic capacity and muscle size. Fitness enthusiasts would vouch for the 'feel good factor' that exercise showers, which is much more than just the satisfaction of achievement. This 'feel-good factor' is spurred by the release of endorphins, known as 'feel-good' hormones, which act as natural mood lifters. Another player in the field is serotonin, a neurotransmitter, commonly termed as the 'happiness hormone'. Exercise stimulates the growth of new brain cells, which in turn boosts the level of serotonin, leading to an improved mood and increased senses of well-being and happiness.

Additionally, exercise enhances cognition by promoting neuroplasticity and neurogenesis. It aids in the creation of new neural connections and boosts cerebral blood period, fueling mental agility, and improving memory and thinking capacity. Multiple studies have even revealed a cutback in the symptoms of numerous mental health conditions including anxiety and depression, endorsing the profound influence of physical fitness on mental well-being.

4.2. Exercise: A Burst of Feel-Good Chemicals

Exercise triggers the brain to dump chemicals like dopamine, norepinephrine, and serotonin in a much higher dosage, setting off the happiness alarm within us. Let's engage in a deeper understanding of these internal bliss makers:

- **Dopamine** is a neurochemical that drives the brain's reward system. When you reach that new fitness milestone, dopamine is the star component of that shot of joy and satisfaction you feel.

- **Serotonin**'s main role is in helping regulate mood, sleep, appetite, and even social behaviour. Low levels of serotonin can lead to depression and anxiety. This is where regular exercise steps in, flooding the brain with this neurotransmitter, and staving off negative mental conditions.

- **Norepinephrine** acts as both a stress hormone and neurotransmitter. It's responsible for the 'fight or flight' response to stressful situations. Proper focus and attention – particularly during those deadlifts and Pilates sessions – require healthy levels of this chemical.

Exercise, hence, acts as a natural mood enhancer, motivating a surge of these chemicals, and leading to a happier, more positive mental state.

4.3. Choosing the Right Exercise for Your Mood Enhancement

All physical activity contributes to an improved mood, but here are some exercises you might want to focus on:

- **Aerobic exercises**: Walking, running, swimming, and cycling are amazing ways to uplift your mood. They help to reduce anxiety and depression, and improve sleep.

- **Yoga and Pilates**: These mind-body exercises improve mental resilience and reduce stress, transforming the outlook towards life into a more positive one.

- **Resistance training**: Lifting weights or body strength exercises can alleviate feelings of depression and foster feelings of empowerment and control.

- **Tai Chi**: This Chinese martial art form reduces stress, boosts mood and even helps deal with chronic conditions like heart disease and arthritis.

Certainly, the most effective exercise is the one you'll stick with. You don't necessarily need to run a marathon to reap the mental health benefits of exercise. The key is to find what you enjoy and make it a part of your routine.

4.4. Ensuring Consistency: Making Fitness a Way of Life

Benefiting from the mental health improvements that come with exercise isn't about working out to the point of exhaustion. Mental well-being blooms from exercising consistently. Start slow and gradually increase your activities. Even a 15-minutes walk can inject your day with a fresh burst of mood-boosting endorphins. Keeping consistency can be challenging in our busy lives, hence integrating exercise into your daily routines or associating it with activities you enjoy can be helpful.

===Conclusion: Enrich Your Life with Exercise

There's no denying the profound influence of physical fitness on mental well-being. When you embrace fitness, not only your physique, but your mind morphs too as it becomes more resilient to stress, anxiety, and other mental health conditions. By regular exercises that trigger a cascade of mood-lifting chemicals, you can plough through negative emotions and foster positivity. As you embark on this invigorating journey to mental health enrichment, remember, every step counts, every time your heart rate increases, you're not just working towards a healthier body, but also a happier mind!

If you have a mental health concern, remember it's always best to reach out to healthcare professionals who can provide you with advice nuanced to your needs and situation. Exercise is a brilliant tool for managing mental well-being, but it doesn't replace professional guidance when needed. So stay active, stay happy, and let's gallop towards good health together!

Chapter 5. Combatting Stress: The Role of Healthy Eating and Regular Exercise

In the swirling storm of our everyday lives, stress is almost an inevitable trial. The moving parts of our daily routines often serve up a hefty serving of stress, leaving us overwhelmed and anxious. But how we respond to this stress makes all the difference. We have two potential sources of solace waiting for us: nutrition and exercise. These lifestyle changes combat stress and offer an effective way to manage our mental well-being.

5.1. Understanding Stress

Before we delve into the remedies, it's important to get acquainted with our culprit. Stress is a normal physiological response occurring when we face challenges or threatening situations. During these events, the body unleashes a cascade of hormones, including adrenaline and cortisol, preparing us for the 'fight or flight' response. Occasional stress is beneficial and keeps us alert. However, chronic stress depletes our mental and physical resources, leading to detrimental effects on our health.

5.2. Consequence of Chronic Stress

Chronic stress, synonymous with our fast-paced lives, does more than just damage our mental health. It disrupts our body's rhythm, leading to compromised immunity and enhanced risk of various physical ailments. These include heart diseases, diabetes, a weakened immune system, and much more. But perhaps the biggest toll it takes is on our mental health, contributing to conditions like anxiety, depression, and a consistent low mood.

5.3. The Role of Nutrition in Stress Management

Maintaining a balanced diet is one of the first steps towards a healthier mind. Various nutrients are required by our brain to produce neurotransmitters, the chemical messengers that regulate our mood and stress response.

For instance, the consumption of complex carbohydrates such as whole grains and vegetables promotes the production of serotonin, a neurotransmitter known for its calming effect. Omega-3 fatty acids, found in fatty fish and flaxseeds, reduce anxiety levels and prevent mood disorders. Vitamins like B-complex and C are vital for the synthesis of neurotransmitters and regulation of stress response, respectively.

Adopting a Mediterranean style diet, high in fruits, vegetables, lean proteins, and healthy fats, is often advocated by nutritionists for its numerous physical and mental health benefits. A 2013 study published in BMC Medicine suggests that following a Mediterranean diet may help prevent the onset of mental health conditions like depression.

It might be tempting to turn to comfort foods - high in fat, sugar, and salt - during stressful times. However, while these foods provide immediate pleasure, they contribute to long-term health issues and exacerbate stress. Learning to nurture your body with good-quality, nutrient-rich food is vital for overall well-being.

5.4. Exercise and Stress Relief: A Biological Perspective

Exercise isn't just about building muscles or staying fit, it's a form of self-care that directly impacts your mental health. When you engage in physical activity, your body produces endorphins or also known as 'feel-good' hormones, a natural mood lifter that also acts as a natural analgesic. Exercise also reduces levels of the body's stress hormones, such as adrenaline and cortisol.

Activities like yoga and tai chi combine physical movement with breath control and meditation, which induces relaxation and reduces stress. Several scientific studies reinforce the idea that regular physical activity lowers anxiety and enhances mood, providing a natural remedy for managing stress.

5.5. Building a Healthy Eating and Exercise Habit: Some Tips

Adopting a new habit isn't easy. It requires consistent efforts towards a specified goal. Here are some tips to help you get started:

1. Start Small: Trying to make a big change all at once can be overwhelming. Start with manageable goals, like adding a piece of fruit to your meal or taking a short walk every day.

2. Consistency is Key: A balanced diet and regular exercise routine are habits that need to be developed over time. Even on days when you don't feel up to it, strive to make healthy choices.

3. Find Activities You Love: Exercise shouldn't be a chore. Find activities that you enjoy, which will make you more likely to keep up with them in the long run.

4. Reach out for Support: Share your fitness journey with others. Join a workout group, cook healthy meals with family, and enlist friends' support to help you stay motivated.

5. Manage Your Expectations: Remember that change doesn't happen overnight. Gains in fitness are gradual and require consistent effort.

Combatting stress in today's world can be a daunting task, but proper nutrition and regular exercise can make it more manageable. By incorporating small changes in your lifestyle, you can gradually build healthier habits, reduce stress, and markedly improve your overall mental well-being. Remember, by taking care of your body, you are also taking care of your mind.

Chapter 6. Food and Mood: Understanding the Gut-Brain Connection

The age-old saying, 'you are what you eat', is not just an adage propounded by our ancestors. Today, scientific research confirms that the food we consume plays a significant role not only in our physical health but also in the state of our mental well-being. This chapter takes you through an enlightening exploration of how our food choices relate to our moods, with special reference to a fascinating phenomenon termed the 'Gut-Brain Connection'.

6.1. The Importance of Nutrition in Mental Health

Diet and emotional well-being may appear to inhabit separate realms. However, in reality, these twin aspects of human life are deeply intertwined. Our diets provide the fuel needed by the brain, the command center of our bodies, which in turn regulates our emotional and mental states.

Certain nutrients directly affect brain function by altering the production of critical neurotransmitters, such as serotonin, dopamine, and norepinephrine. These biochemicals help dictate our mood, energy levels, sleep patterns, concentration, and overall cognitive function.

For example, foods rich in Omega-3 fatty acids, such as wild salmon and walnuts, promote the production of serotonin, often referred to as the 'happy hormone'. While low levels of serotonin are linked with depression, higher levels often lead to better moods and overall mental well-being.

6.2. The Gut-Brain Axis: How Your Gut Communicates with Your Brain

Our understanding of nutrition-related influences on mental health took a quantum leap with the discovery of the Gut-Brain Axis. This bidirectional communication highway links our central nervous system (comprising the brain and spinal cord) with the enteric nervous system (the nervous system of our gastrointestinal tract).

Scientific research has shown that our gastrointestinal (GI) tract – often referred to as our second brain – is not solely responsible for digestion. This seemingly low-key bodily function also houses approximately 70% of our immune system, and it's where an intricate interaction between our gut microbiome (microscopic bacteria, viruses, fungi, etc., that live inside our gut) and our brain takes place.

Our gut microbiome performs many functions, including nutrient absorption, immune response regulation, and production of certain vitamins such as K and B12. But the most mind-boggling role it plays is probably the production of key neurotransmitters, including an estimated 90% of our serotonin!

Based on this understanding, it's clear that a healthy, well-functioning gut can contribute positively to our mental health, indicating a powerful new way of understanding disorders like depression, anxiety, and stress.

6.3. Foods That Fuel Your Gut and Your Mind

Recognizing the significance of gut health in mental well-being can be empowering, showing us a curative path that begins right from our kitchen. Here are some foods and food groups known to foster a healthy gut microbiome and, by extension, uplift mental health:

1. Whole grains: Foods such as oats, brown rice, and barley are rich in dietary fiber – a vital food source for our gut bacteria. The digestion of fiber leads to the production of short-chain fatty acids which have been shown to promote brain health.

2. Fermented Foods: Foods like yogurt, kimchi, and sauerkraut are not just tasty; they are also probiotic powerhouses that can help boost the number of good bacteria in your gut.

3. Fruits and vegetables: These are rich in antioxidants and fibers – substances that positively affect the diversity of our gut bacteria.

4. Lean proteins: Foods like fish, chicken breast, and tofu provide us with amino acids necessary to create neurotransmitters.

The participation of food in shaping our mental health opens a range of possibilities to empower ourselves. This knowledge harnesses the potential of breaking free from the clutches of disorders stemming from mental unrest, simply by making conscious choices about what's on our plate.

6.4. Conclusion

Understanding the intricate relationship between food, gut health, and mental well-being can revolutionize the way we approach our diets and overall lifestyle. As we pay heed to fostering a healthful diet and regular exercise, we simultaneously open the doors to a better mental state.

Nutrition is not just about keeping physical ailments at bay, but it also ushers in an upliftment of our mental state or a more joyful, lively existence. With this knowledge, each one of us holds the power not just to nourish our bodies, but also our minds, through conscious, mindful eating.

In the end, remember this all-important lesson: Your gut health is a reflection of your mental health in more ways than you may have imagined. Over time, taking care of your gut health can lead to an enhanced state of mental well-being, allowing for increased productivity, a more positive outlook, and a better quality of life.

Chapter 7. Neuroplasticity: How Nutrition and Exercise Reshape Your Brain

Hippocrates, the ancient Greek physician and 'father of medicine', wisely stated, "Let thy food be thy medicine, and thy medicine be thy food." Interestingly, this applies as much to our brains as to our bodies. In recent years, neuroscientists have uncovered the fascinating ability of the brain to change its structure, function, and chemistry in response to experience, behavior, environment, and neural processes. This phenomenon is known as neuroplasticity.

7.1. The Fundamentals of Neuroplasticity

The human brain is not a rigid organ, fixed in its ways. Instead, it is remarkably dynamic, continually changing and adapting in response to new experiences, learning, and challenges. These changes are driven by our activities, what we perceive, feel, and do. And more importantly, what we eat and how we approach fitness.

Neuroplasticity is based on two main principles: 'Neurons that fire together, wire together', meaning that the frequent activation of certain neural pathways strengthens the connections, and 'use it or lose it', underlining the fact that neural connections deteriorate with disuse. Both of these principles emphasize the interactive and malleable nature of our brains.

7.2. Nutrition and Neuroplasticity

From providing energy to serving as building blocks for brain cells, the food we consume plays a critical role in influencing brain health.

Essential nutrients like omega-3 fatty acids, resveratrol, curcumin, and vitamins B12 and D are particularly vital for promoting neuroplasticity. Omega-3s, for instance, found in fatty fish, help reduce brain inflammation and promote new brain cell formation. Resveratrol, a potent antioxidant found in red wine and grapes, potentially strengthens the blood-brain barrier, protecting the brain from harmful substances. Foods rich in curcumin, like turmeric, and those beaming with vitamin B12, greatly contribute to nerve health and synaptic plasticity.

On the contrary, consuming excessive amounts of refined sugars, unhealthy fats, and processed foods can potentially disrupt neuronal connections in the brain. This kind of diet is also known to affect the microbiome-gut-brain axis, leading to elevated levels of inflammation and oxidative stress, which over time, can impair cognitive health and overall brain function.

7.3. Exercise and Neuroplasticity

Physical exercise, specifically aerobic exercise, has a profound impact on your brain's health and neuroplasticity. Regular exercise increases brain-derived neurotrophic factor (BDNF), a protein that supports the survival of existing neurons, encourages the growth of new neurons and synapses, and improves cognition.

Exercise also enhances the brain's plasticity by stimulating neurogenesis (the creation of new neurons) in the hippocampus, an area of the brain critical for learning, memory, and mood regulation. Moreover, it helps release endorphins, the body's "feel-good" hormones, thus promoting a sense of wellbeing and contentment.

Walking, running, cycling, swimming, or any form of aerobic exercise can support neuroplasticity. The key is to choose activities that you enjoy, making it more likely that you'll stick with them over the long term.

7.4. The Correlation Between Nutrition, Exercise, and Mental Well-being

When we nourish our bodies with good food and regular exercise, it's not just our physical health that benefits. Our mental well-being can also greatly improve. And this is where the intricate relationship between nutrition, fitness, and neuroplasticity comes into play.

A diet fueling neuroplasticity, paired with regular physical activity, can help shape our brain's structure in a way that promotes cognitive clarity, alertness, and positive mood states. It allows our brain to adapt more effectively to new information and changes, thereby enhancing our ability to learn, solve problems, make decisions, cope with stress, and connect with others. So, to put Hippocrates' words into the context of brain health, "May the choices that we make in food and exercise be our brain's medicine."

7.5. Making Mindful Lifestyle Choices

Undoubtedly, nurturing our brain's plasticity, akin to shaping a lump of clay, requires conscious effort. However, the rewards of those efforts are immense. From sharpening the mind, increasing our ability to learn and adapt, to alleviating stress, and fostering happiness - what's on our plates and how much we move can create ripples in the pond of mental well-being.

A diet teeming with varied, nutrient-dense whole foods, coupled with a commitment to regular exercise, is a foundation for excellent mental health. The journey toward improved cognitive well-being begins with making mindful lifestyle choices. Let's start nurturing our brain's plasticity and, as a result, our mental well-being with every bite and every step we take!

Remember, mental well-being is not a destination; it's an ongoing journey of self-nourishment and self-discovery. The next time you sit down for a meal, remind yourself: You are not just eating; you are nourishing your brain. And the next time you procrastinate over exercising, remember: You aren't just moving; you are reshaping your brain.

Our power to enhance neuroplasticity through nutrition and exercise is a form of self-care that indeed impacts every facet of life. As we sculpt our brains through these healthy habits, we carve a path to improved cognition, increased resilience, and overall mental well-being – steering us closer to the essence of good health - happiest mind in the healthiest body. Let us embrace this power, for it's never too late to begin.

Remember, enhancing neuroplasticity is no quick fix. It's a lifestyle commitment. But when you start seeing how powerful these changes can be – in your cognition, emotion regulation, stress resilience, and overall happiness – you will find strength in the journey. After all, life is a continuous quest for growth and adaptation. And our brains, incredible in their neuroplasticity, are our allies in this relentless pursuit.

Alchemy might not be real, but we have something even more magic - our brain's intrinsic capacity to transform and adapt. So, let's fuel it with the right nutrition, keep it active with regular exercise, and behold the magic of neuroplasticity, propelling us towards holistic well-being.

Remember, brain health is achievable. And each step we take, each bite we eat, moves us closer to that goal. Because, the truth is, it's not just about living longer. It's about living better, thinking clearer, feeling happier. And that begins in the brain.

So, let's start shaping that ultimate piece of art - our brain, with the beautiful tools of nutrition and fitness. And let's align our journey with profound words by Norman Cousins, "The human brain is not just a problem-solving organ. It is the highest form of a pleasure-generating apparatus."

Indeed, the capability of our brains to reshape and refine itself underscores the remarkable potential that lies within us, a potential unleashed through healthy eating and physical exercise. Let's relish this empowering journey of discovering our minds' full capability, one neuron at a time, and let us all strive to make our brains the epitome of health, cognitive sharpness, and happiness. You have the power to create the best version of your brain. It all starts with a decision - a decision to maintain the right mind-body balance through the perfect blend of enriching nutrition and invigorating physical activity. Embrace the journey; cherish the transformation.

Chapter 8. Break the Norm: Fun Workouts for Mental Stimulus

The cemented perception about staying fit typically takes us to a mind frame of lifting weights and doing cardio, but let's take a different route to stimulate our minds and bodies! Think dance-offs, rafting, outdoor Pilates, or even hula hooping. Yes, you read it right. Fun workouts simply attempt to incorporate "play" into the otherwise repetitive and monotonous exercise regimen, providing both physical and mental stimulus.

8.1. The Power of Fun Workouts

Before getting on to the real stuff, let's first understand the science behind it. As we engage ourselves in a fun physical activity, our bodies release chemicals known as endorphins, neurotransmitters responsible for feelings of happiness and euphoria. But did you know that they act as natural painkillers too? These chemicals interact with the receptors in your brain to reduce the perception of pain and deliver a positive feeling in the body, similar to morphine.

According to the American Psychological Association (APA), any form of physical activity can act as a stress-reliever, improving the way our bodies work with stress chemicals and balancing our moods over time.

8.2. It's not just Cardio!

CrossFit and spin classes can sure pump up adrenaline but aren't the only source of cardio. Activities like skipping, hula hooping, or pursuits like belly dancing provide burn calories while you're at play.

Here's how these non-traditional workouts stimulate your body and mind.

1. **Hula Hooping**: This isn't just for kids! Integrating a hula hoop into your routine could help improve balance and flexibility, along with providing a great cardio workout. And it can burn as many calories as step aerobics or a brisk walk!

2. **Skipping**: Remember how much fun it was to jump rope on your school playground? Skipping indeed works as an excellent cardio with the added element of fun, enhancing your body agility, quickness, and foot coordination.

3. **Belly Dancing**: An excellent form of cardio, Belly dancing, is more than just a fun shake. Ancient art that initially had a spiritual significance, it boosts body positivity and enhances lower body strength.

8.3. Exercise your Brain with Chessboxing

Chessboxing – yes, it's exactly what it looks like, chess and boxing mashed together in a hybrid sport – is a fantastic way of catering to both the physical and mental stimulus. This unusual sport, first coined by a French artist Enki Bilal in his comic book "Froid Equateur," requires you to exercise both physically and mentally. You'll find yourself quickly switching from attacking with rooks and knights to throwing jabs and uppercuts in the boxing ring.

8.4. Laugh Out Loud with Laughter Yoga

Laughter Yoga, a fusion of yogic breathing practices with laughter exercises, promises health and happiness. Brought to popular notice by the Indian physician Madan Kataria, it engages people in spontaneous laughter, ultimately leading to the release of dopamine, a chemical in the brain which triggers a sense of pleasure. It improves oxygen supply, boosts mood, reduces stress, and fortifies your immune system.

8.5. Why not try a Colour Run?

Running - a strenuous, monotonous exercise, behold! Here's a color run for you. Also known as the 'happiest 5k on the planet,' these runs aren't timed. It's not about who comes first or last but about having fun. And as you reach the finish line, you're welcomed with a color burst of a party, creating memories in technicolor.

8.6. Virtual Reality Workouts

Yes, we are living in the age of technology, so why not bring it to our workouts! Virtual Reality workouts can turn your dull 30-minute workout into an adventurous trip. Fight off zombies or punch to the tunes of music, you can try them all! It's not just exciting but it also helps you with stress management and enhancing your cognitive skills.

These aren't just workouts, they are experiences! The whole idea behind fun workouts is to break the perception of monotonous, strenuous gym routines alone constituting fitness. It's time to shift the focus to what feels good instead of what looks good. It's time to take charge, relieve stress, and most importantly, have fun while we do it, because isn't that what being healthy should be all about? Choose your kind of fun and let's get started!

Chapter 9. Making Fitness and Nutrition a Habit: Strategies for Successful Implementation

In order to optimize mental well-being, it's crucial to instill a genuine commitment to fitness and nutrition in everyday life. This chapter provides strategies for making fitness and nutrition a habit for lasting improvements in mental health.

9.1. Understanding the Link Between Fitness, Nutrition, and Mental Well-being

Scientific research has repeatedly underscored the correlation between physical activity, a balanced diet, and improved mental well-being. Exercise increases the production of endorphins, 'feel-good' chemicals in the brain, combating stress, anxiety, and depression. Similarly, a nutritionally-rich diet provides the essential nutrients your brain needs for optimal function, promoting cognitive function, mood, and overall mental well-being.

9.2. Establishing Mindful Eating Habits

Mindful eating involves developing awareness of your hunger and satiety cues, recognizing your emotional responses to food, and understanding the nutritional value of what you eat. The following strategies can help you foster mindful eating.

1. Create a conducive eating environment: Minimize distractions during meals to focus on the food and your body's responses.

2. Develop a meal schedule: Regular meal times can prevent overeating and ensure you maintain optimal nutrient intake.

3. Practise portion control: Use smaller plates to help manage portion sizes, and refrain from second helpings.

4. Listen to your body: Train yourself to recognize when you are genuinely hungry and when you've had enough.

9.3. Incorporating Regular Physical Activity

Incorporating regular activity into your daily routine doesn't mean spending grueling hours at the gym; rather, it involves making little changes that add up to an active lifestyle. Use these tips to gradually include more physical activities in your routine.

1. Choose activities you enjoy: You're more likely to stick with activities you find fun and enjoyable.

2. Combine physical activity with social interaction: Go for a walk with a friend or join a sports club to kill two birds with one stone.

3. Regular, shorter sessions: If lengthy workouts seem daunting, aim for regular, shorter bursts of activity.

9.4. Overcoming Obstacles to Fitness and Nutrition

Let's explore strategies to address common barriers preventing us from adopting healthy eating and fitness habits.

1. Time management: Plan ahead for meals, workout sessions, etc., to ensure that they fit into your schedule.

2. Prioritize: Assess your commitments. If fitness and nutrition are important for your well-being, dedicate time to them.

3. Build a support system: Enlist the help of friends, partners, and family to help you stay motivated.

9.5. Developing a Mindset for Lifestyle Change

A successful lifestyle change is rooted in a positive and committed mindset. It involves:

1. Set realistic goals: Setting achievable, small, incremental goals can empower you to overcome challenges.

2. Embrace self-compassion: Understand that slip-ups happen; it's your ability to bounce back that matters.

9.6. Fitness and Nutrition for All Ages

Finally, remember that maintaining fitness and nutrition isn't limited by age:

1. Young Adults: Encourage playful physical activity, cultivate an enjoyment for a variety of healthy foods.

2. Adults: Find activities that you enjoy and make them part of your routine. Have a balanced diet.

3. Seniors: Try low-impact exercises. Eat nutrient-dense foods.

By integrating these strategies, we can develop a successful link between fitness, nutrition, and mental well-being, leading to significant, long-lasting improvements in our mental health.

Chapter 10. Achieving Balance: A Holistic Approach to Mental Well-being

Balancing the scales of life isn't easy in our fast-paced, stress-laden society. Nevertheless, achieving equilibrium, especially regarding mental health, is essential for functioning optimally. Many have found solace in the path of holistic wellness, an approach that encompasses physical, mental, and spiritual health. As an integral part of this journey, two components - nutrition and fitness - play pivotal roles.

10.1. How Nutrition Influences Mental Well-being

Many of us have experienced the rush of happiness after enjoying our favorite meal, but there's much more to the food-mood equation than meets the eye. Nutrition directly and indirectly impacts our mental health through complex biochemical processes.

Consider the brain, our body's mastermind, which oversees countless physical and emotional processes. Despite its integral role, it represents only 2% of our body weight. Intriguingly, it consumer a whopping 20% of our daily calorie intake, demonstrating the immense energy requirement for maintaining our brain's functionality.

Research suggests that certain nutrients like Omega-3 fatty acids, B-vitamins, and antioxidants play a crucial role in brain health. These nutrients aid in neurological processes, membrane fluidity, and protecting against oxidative stress, which could potentially lead to standard mental health disorders such as depression.

In essence, what we eat can significantly influence our mental well-being. A balanced diet rich in these essential nutrients can aid in maintaining optimal mental health, paving the way for enhanced cognition, improved mood, and reduced stress levels.

10.2. Fitness: The Physical Route To Mental Well-being

While the role of nutrition is paramount, fitness holds equal importance for maintaining mental well-being. Engaging in regular physical activity exerts a protective influence on the brain. Cardiovascular exercises increase blood flow to the brain, delivering essential nutrients and oxygen. As a result, such workouts boost cognitive function and reduce depressive symptoms.

Furthermore, exercise is a great stress-buster. It encourages the release of endorphins - the body's natural 'feel-good' chemicals that help induce feelings of happiness. Regular workouts can lead to improved self-esteem and sleep quality, both of which have direct links to our mental health. Fitness is not just about weight management or physical attractiveness; it's a stepping stone towards enhancing mental fortitude.

10.3. Merging The Two: A Holistic Approach

Understanding the individual impacts of nutrition and fitness on mental well-being paves the way for a holistic approach involving their integration. After all, maintaining mental health is not a one-track endeavor. Rather, it encompasses various aspects of our lifestyles, and both nutrition and fitness are significant players in this arena.

Combining healthy eating habits with a regular workout regimen can yield optimal mental well-being. Nutrient-rich food fuels the body for physical activities, while workouts alleviate stress and promote overall wellbeing. In this way, nutrition and fitness can work symbiotically to enhance mental health.

Moreover, consistency is key. Following a specific diet or workout plan for a brief period can yield benefits, but maintaining these habits long-term leads to enduring mental health improvements. Remember, transformation doesn't occur overnight but is a lifelong journey.

10.4. The Vortex Of Mindfulness

Another significant aspect of a holistic approach to mental well-being is mindfulness. Incorporating mindful practices into nutrition and fitness routines can provide an added layer of mental health benefits.

During meals, mindful eating involves completely focusing on the meal, appreciating the food's flavors, textures, and aromas. On the fitness front, mindful exercises such as yoga and Tai Chi connect the body and mind, promoting relaxation and stress management. Mindfulness is not merely an activity; it's a higher quality of attention, encouraging us to live in the present moment and instilling a sense of peace and tranquility — key facets of mental well-being.

10.5. Breaking Down The Barriers

Embarking on a holistic wellness journey may seem daunting at first. However, it's all about breaking down the process into manageable portions. Start slow, make small changes, gradually moving towards the larger goal.

The initial phase might be challenging, but consistency, perseverance, and patience are the pillars supporting this journey. It might take time, but the invincible mental fortress built through consistency will be worth every drop of sweat spent and every bite of healthy food consumed.

In conclusion, the path to mental well-being is an enriching journey that syncs the physical, mental, and spiritual elements of life. Proper nutrition and regular fitness, when adopted holistically, form an unshakeable foundation for mental well-being. As we advance on this journey, remember that it's not about reaching a destination but about fostering long-standing, sustainable changes that bring you a sense of overall happiness and fulfillment.

Chapter 11. Moving Forward: Embracing the Future of Nutrition and Fitness for Mental Health

As we navigate the labyrinth of life, our wellness, particularly mental health, becomes of paramount significance. Embracing nutrition and fitness stands as an inspiring proposition, as they are not merely tools for physical well-being, but potent instruments fostering mental health.

Chapter 12. Understanding the Interplay

Let's begin by acknowledging the interplay between nutrition, fitness and mental health. The chemistry of our brains, and hence our moods, thoughts, and stress levels, are influenced by the foods we consume. Our central nervous system requires a steady stream of nutrients to function optimally. Deficiencies can give rise to symptoms ranging from fatigue to more severe conditions like depression.

Conversely, physical exercise boosts mood-enhancing chemicals, supports neural growth and fosters calmness. It equips us better to handle stress, enhances cognitive abilities, improves sleep and uplifts self-image.

Chapter 13. Nutrition For Mental Health

Assuming a more nutritionally rich diet isn't just about avoiding processed foods rich in fat or sugar. Rather, it's about promoting foods containing nutrients known to support good mental health.

13.1. Brain Boosting Foods

Whole grains, rich in carbohydrates, produce glucose slowly, facilitating better concentration. Foods high in protein - lean meat, poultry, eggs, tofu - break down into amino acids, several of which are essential for mental vigour.

Foods rich in essential omega-3 fats (such as oily fish, flaxseeds, and walnuts) and mono-unsaturated fats (avocados, almonds, peanuts, and olives) are essential for the brain's structure and function.

Ensuring a diet rich in fruits and vegetables provides the nutrients and antioxidants necessary to maintain and repair cells in the body and brain.

13.2. Supplements and Mental Health

While diet stands at the core of our mental well-being, in some instances, certain supplements can bolster the nutritional environment of the brain. Fish oil supplements rich in EPA and DHA are beneficial for mental health. Other important supplements include Vitamin D, B-complex vitamins and Magnesium.

Always consider supplements as a secondary measure, ideally with guidance from a healthcare professional.

Chapter 14. Fitness For Mental Health

While the correlation between physical fitness and mental health might not be as instantly apparent as with nutrition, there is an array of research highlighting the powerful impact of physical activity on our mental well-being.

14.1. Psychological and Neural Benefits

Physical exercise reduces stress hormones and increases the production of endorphins — chemicals in the brain acting as mood elevators. Regular exercise can contribute to improved mood, increased energy levels and better sleep, all of which have profoundly positive effects on mental health.

Fitness activities stimulate the growth of new neural connections, leading to improved cognitive function. Exercising also enhances the brain's ability to change and adapt, a process known as neuroplasticity — vital in maintaining and improving mental health.

14.2. Finding the Right Fitness Regime

The variety and sheer abundance of fitness practices might seem overwhelming at first. The key lies in personalising your fitness regime to align with your lifestyle, preferences and goals. Be it yoga, brisk walking, strength training, swimming or playing a sport, find what resonates with you.

Ensure regularity rather than intensity and be consistent. Remember, even a little movement is better than none.

Chapter 15. Practicing Mindfulness For Mental Health

Unifying nutrition and fitness is the overarching principle of mindfulness — being aware and making conscious choices regarding what you eat and how you move.

Mindfully eating means enjoying the food, being aware not just of the physical sensations of hunger and satiety, but also the sensorial experience of flavours, textures, aromas. This approach enables us to foster a healthier relationship with food and avoid mindless gorging or emotional eating.

Moreover, embedding mindfulness in your exercise routine can amplify its benefits. It helps you engage fully with the physical activity and get in touch with your body, fostering self-awareness and self-acceptance while relieving stress.

Chapter 16. Embracing the Future of Nutrition and Fitness

Investing in our nutrition and fitness is investing in our mental health, a prevalent theme in our current society. It is incredibly empowering to realise the control we can take over our mental health by making mindful choices about our food and our physical activities.

As we move forward, it's crucial to remember that sustainable lifestyle alterations rather than transient fixes make the difference. The trick lies in harnessing these principles in ways that blend into our lifestyles seamlessly.

Nutrition and fitness for mental health is a journey, a continuous learning and adapting process. Along the way, remember to be patient with yourself and celebrate the tiny victories.

As you integrate these insights into your life, know that every step you take towards healthier nutrition and fitness practices is a step towards improved mental health. Here's to a healthier, happier future!

www.ingramcontent.com/pod-product-compliance
Lightning Source LLC
Chambersburg PA
CBHW071005260726
48661CB00007B/2806